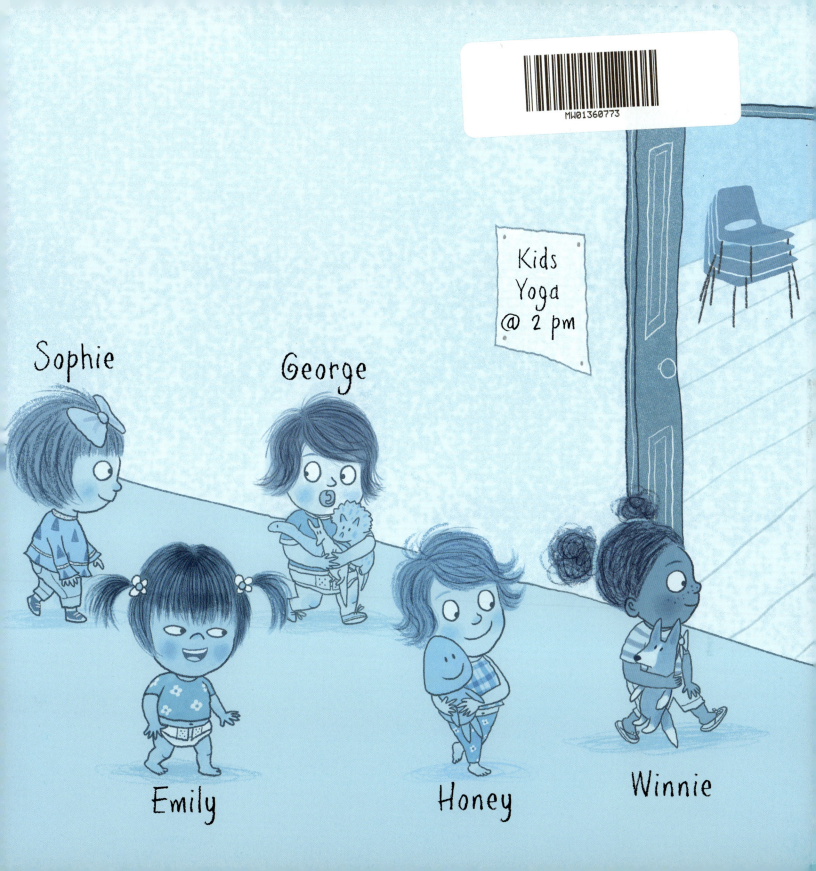

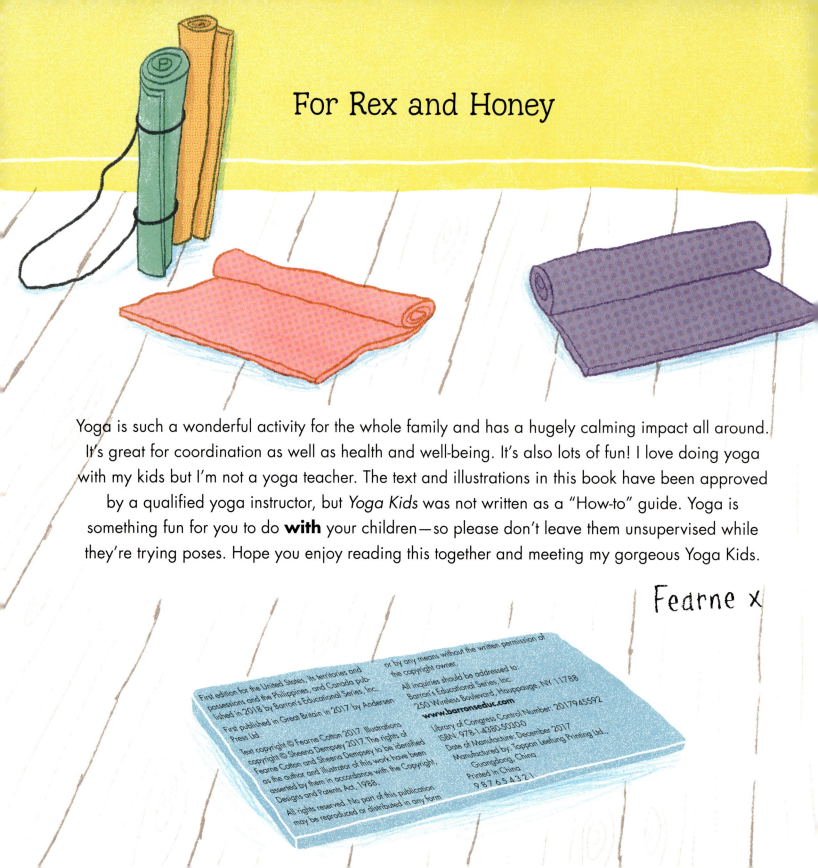

For Rex and Honey

Yoga is such a wonderful activity for the whole family and has a hugely calming impact all around. It's great for coordination as well as health and well-being. It's also lots of fun! I love doing yoga with my kids but I'm not a yoga teacher. The text and illustrations in this book have been approved by a qualified yoga instructor, but *Yoga Kids* was not written as a "How-to" guide. Yoga is something fun for you to do **with** your children—so please don't leave them unsupervised while they're trying poses. Hope you enjoy reading this together and meeting my gorgeous Yoga Kids.

Fearne x

First edition for the United States, its territories and possessions and the Philippines, and Canada published in 2018 by Barron's Educational Series, Inc.

First published in Great Britain in 2017 by Andersen Press Ltd.

Text copyright © Fearne Cotton 2017. Illustrations copyright © Sheena Dempsey 2017. The rights of Fearne Cotton and Sheena Dempsey to be identified as the author and illustrator of this work have been asserted by them in accordance with the Copyright, Designs and Patents Act, 1988.

All rights reserved. No part of this publication may be reproduced or distributed in any form or by any means without the written permission of the copyright owner.

All inquiries should be addressed to:
Barron's Educational Series, Inc.
250 Wireless Boulevard, Hauppauge, NY 11788
www.barronseduc.com

Library of Congress Control Number: 2017945592
ISBN: 978-1-4380-5030-0
Date of Manufacture: December 2017
Manufactured by: Toppan Leefung Printing Ltd.,
Guangdong, China
Printed in China
9 8 7 6 5 4 3 2 1

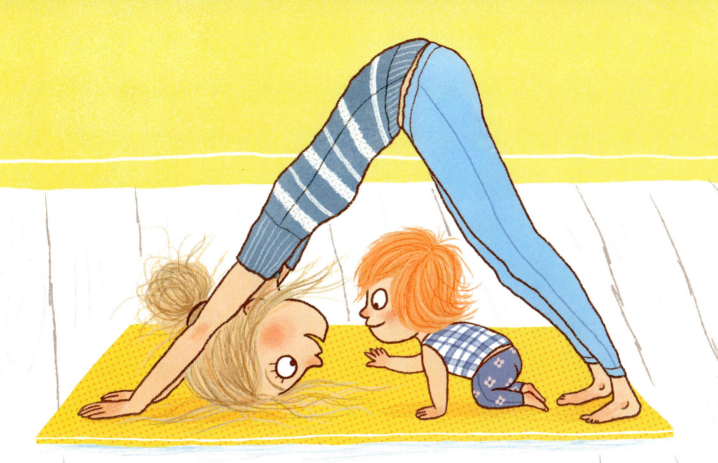

FEARNE COTTON
Yoga Kids

Illustrated by Sheena Dempsey

BARRON'S

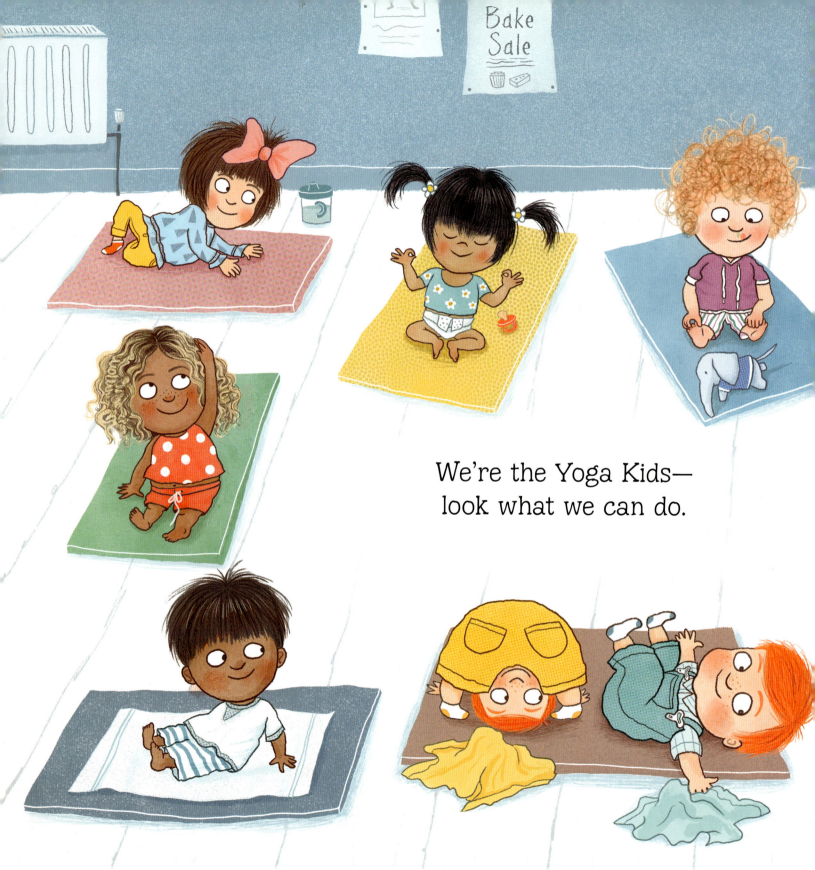

We're the Yoga Kids—
look what we can do.

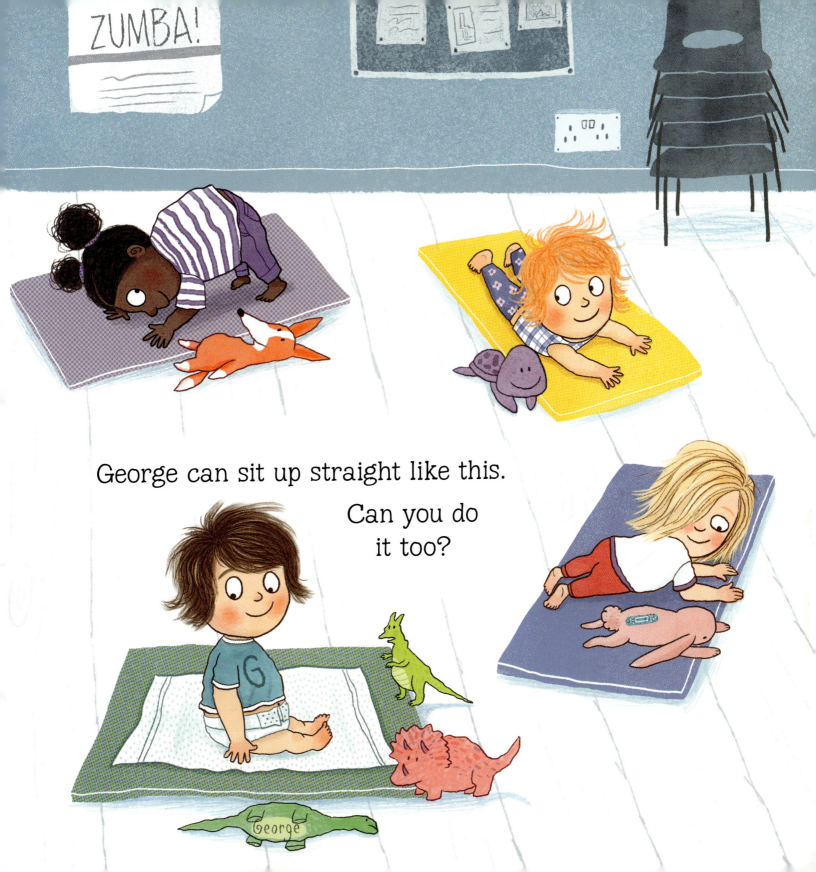
George can sit up straight like this. Can you do it too?

This is little Honey,
she likes to touch her nose.

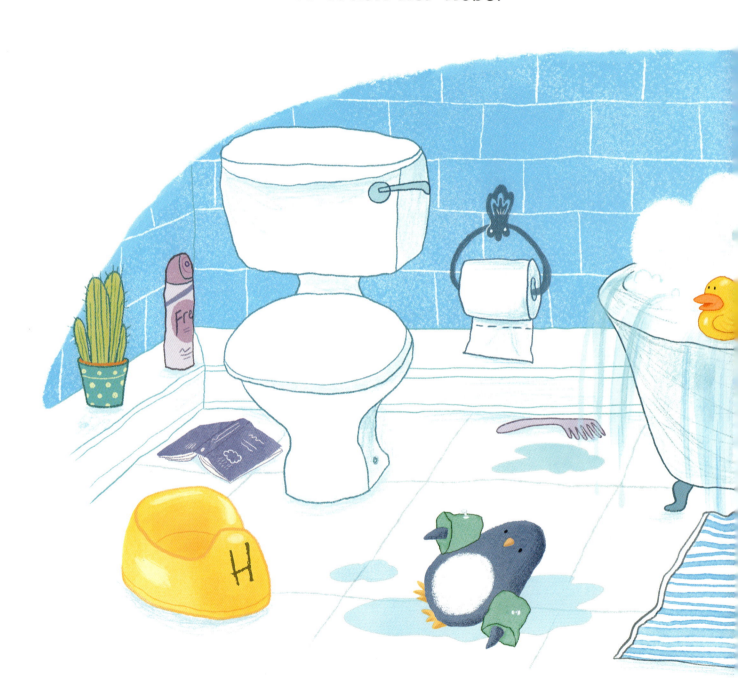

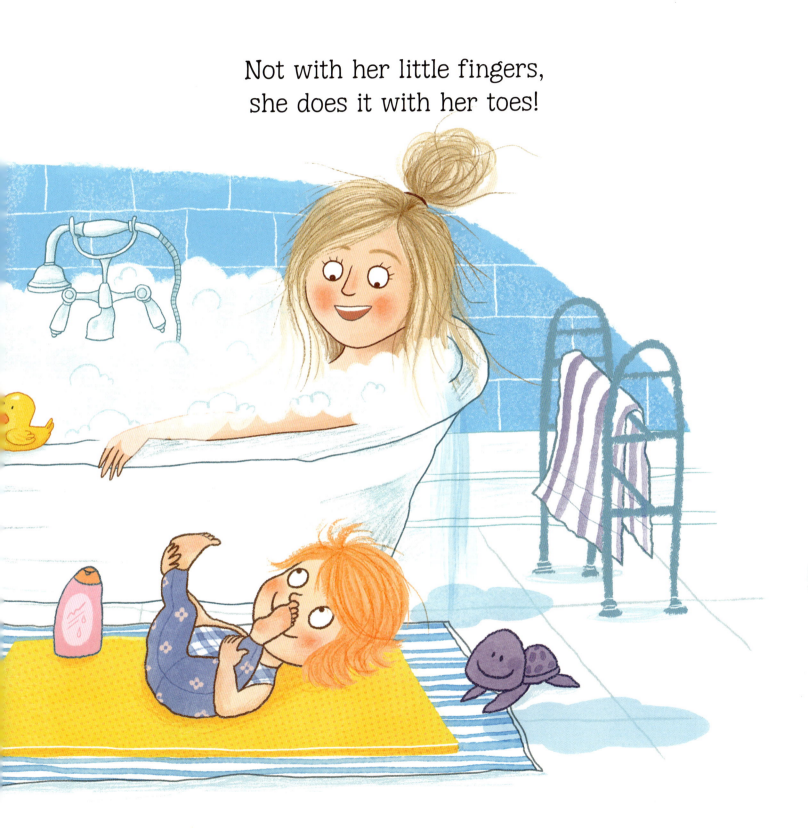

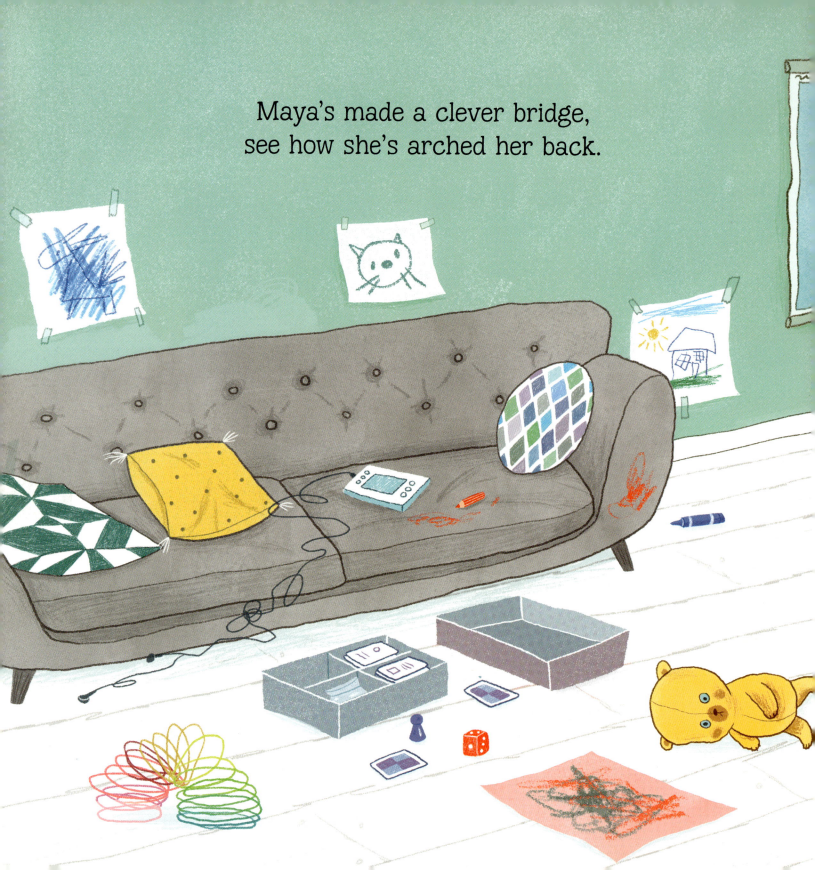
Maya's made a clever bridge,
see how she's arched her back.

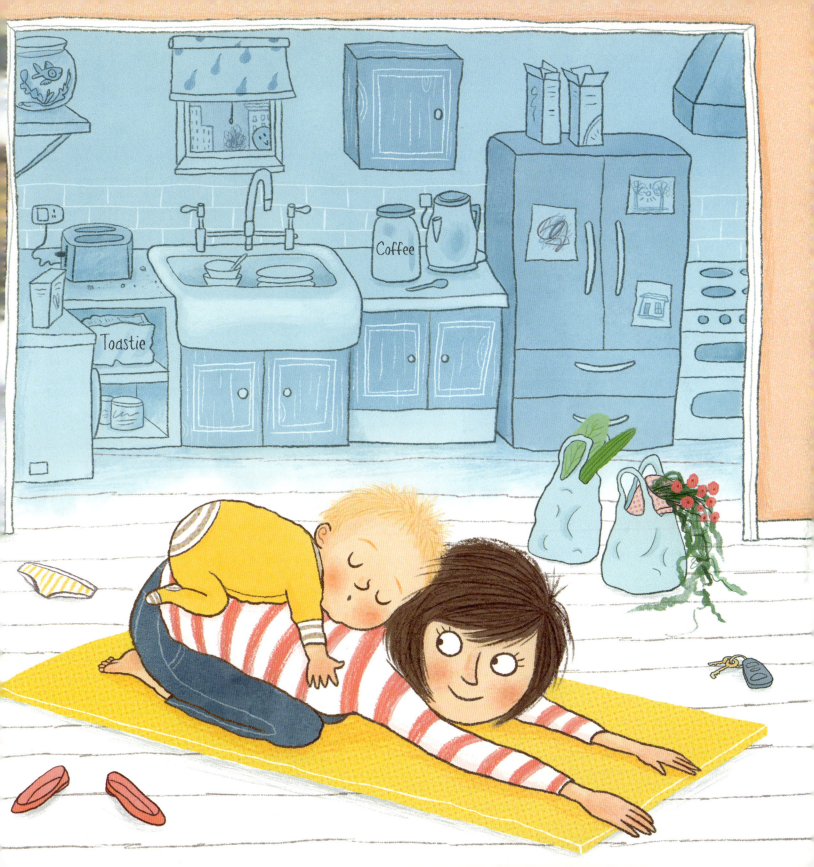

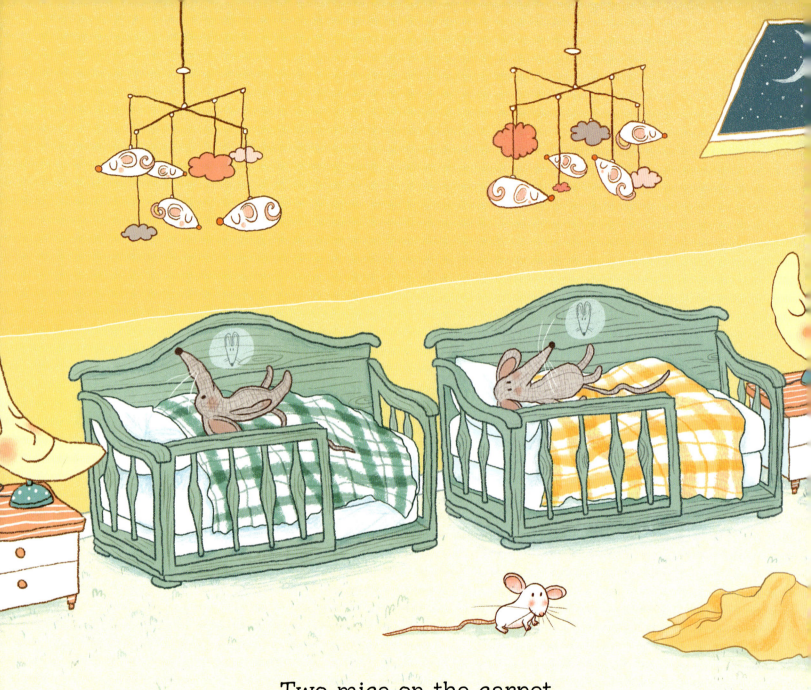

Two mice on the carpet,
curled up so, so tight.
It's Tom and Sam in dormouse pose—
they'll sleep well tonight.

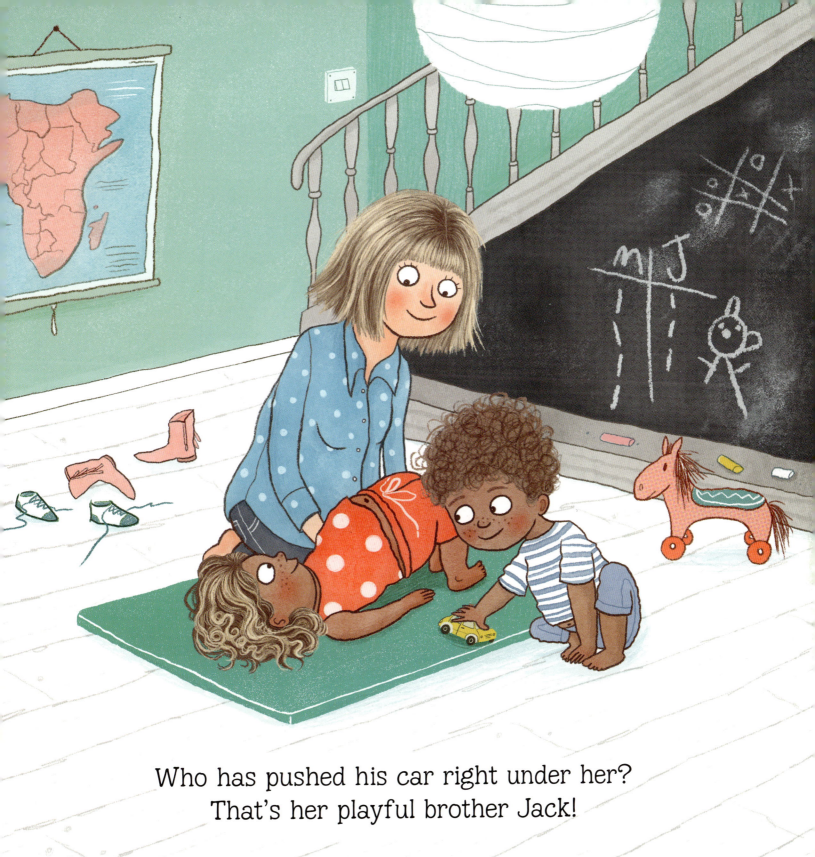

Who has pushed his car right under her?
That's her playful brother Jack!

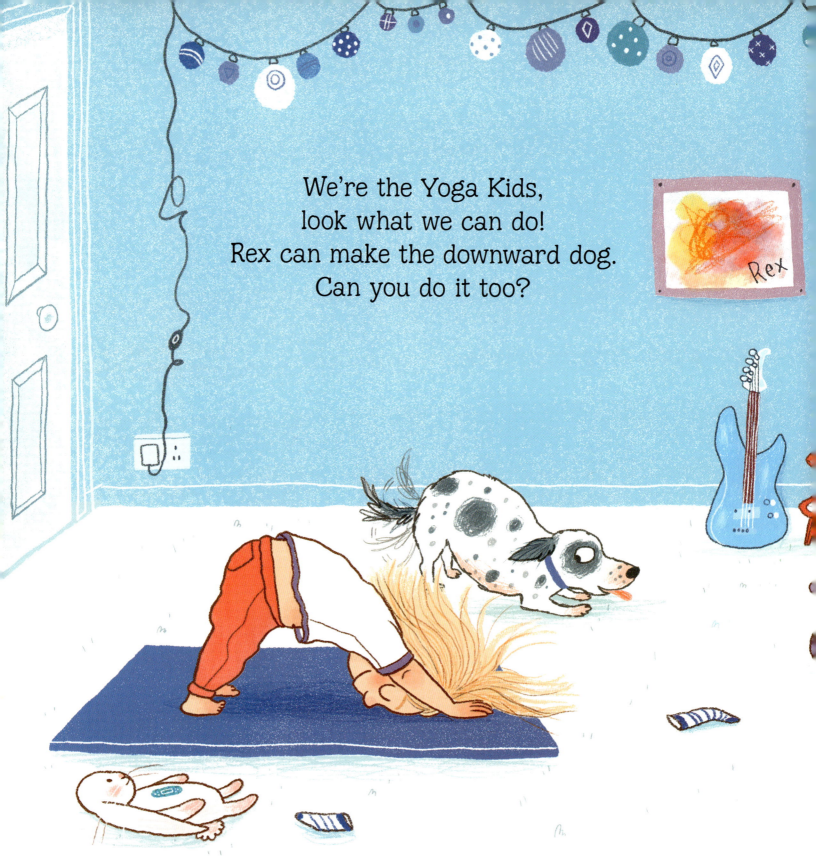

We're the Yoga Kids,
look what we can do!
Rex can make the downward dog.
Can you do it too?

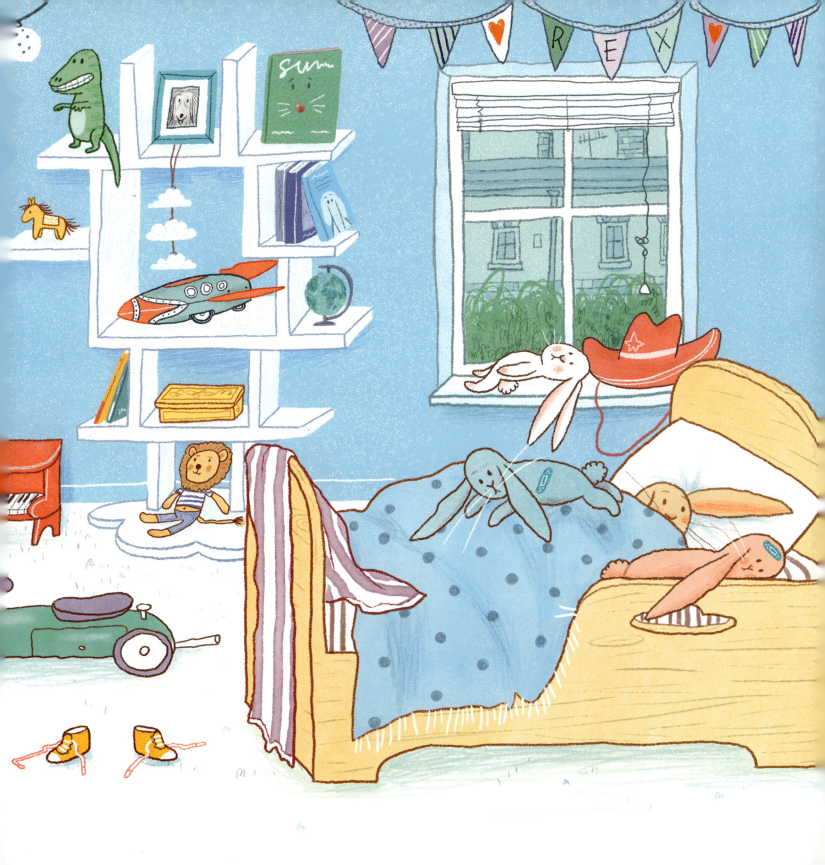

Sophie and her mommy have had a really bad day.

Ben was sick...

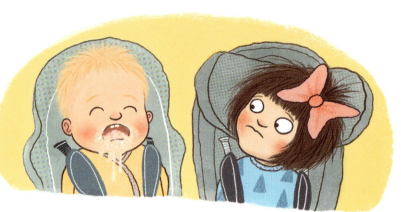

the car broke down...

and then Tiggs, the cat, ran away.

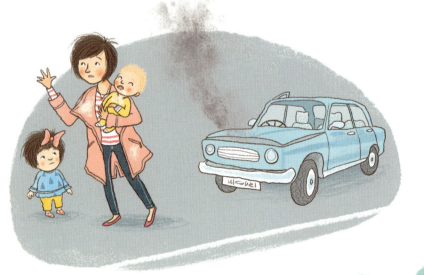

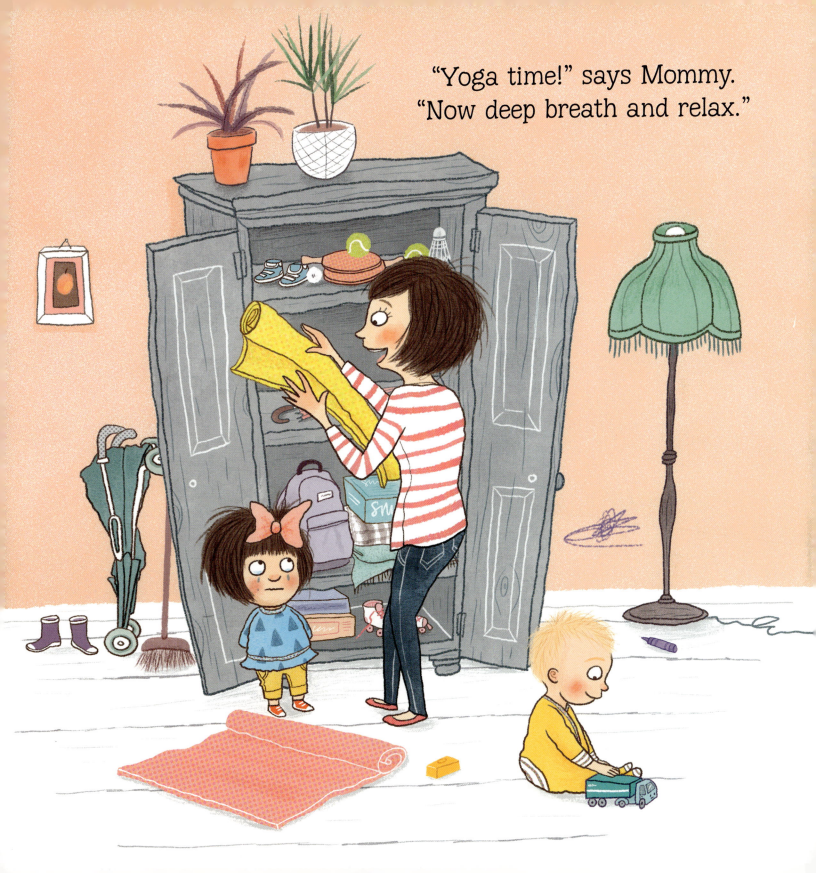

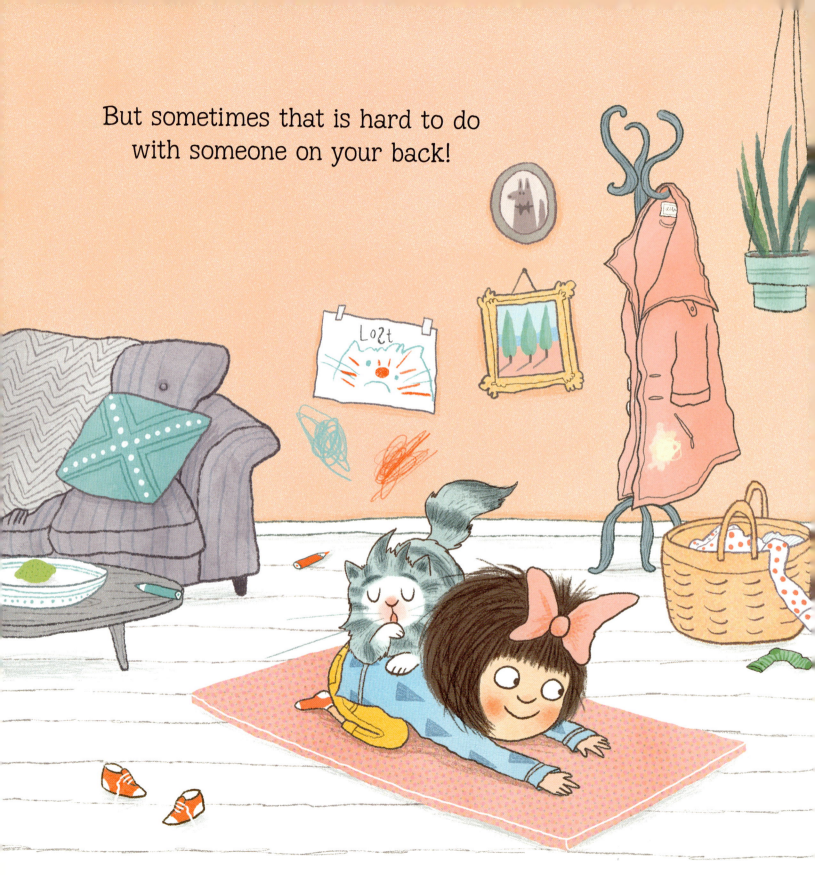

But sometimes that is hard to do with someone on your back!

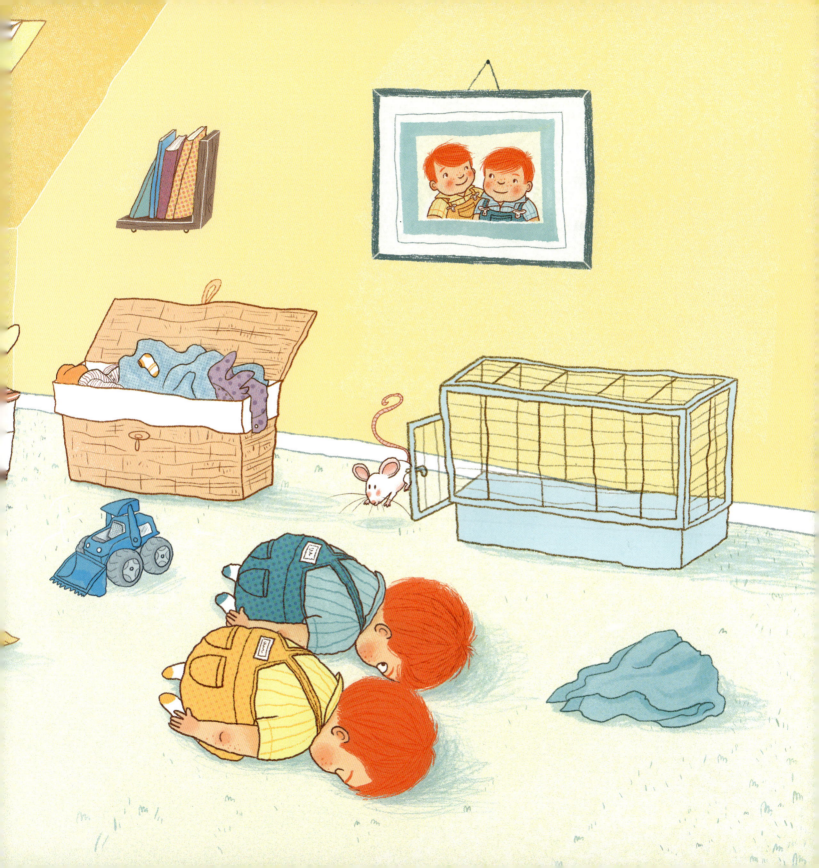

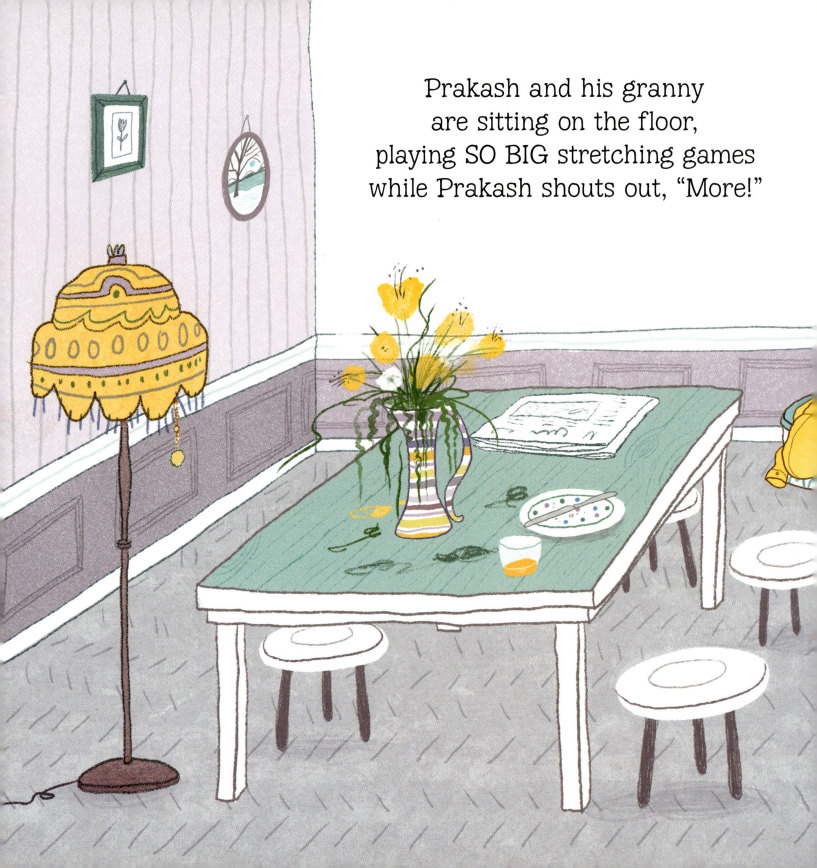
Prakash and his granny are sitting on the floor, playing SO BIG stretching games while Prakash shouts out, "More!"

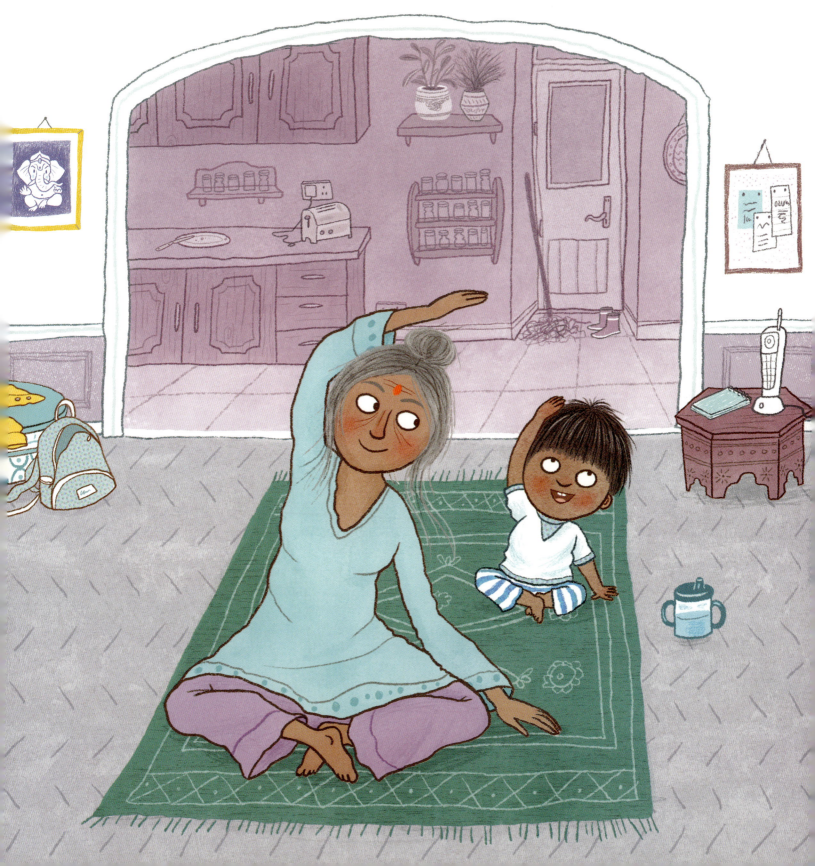

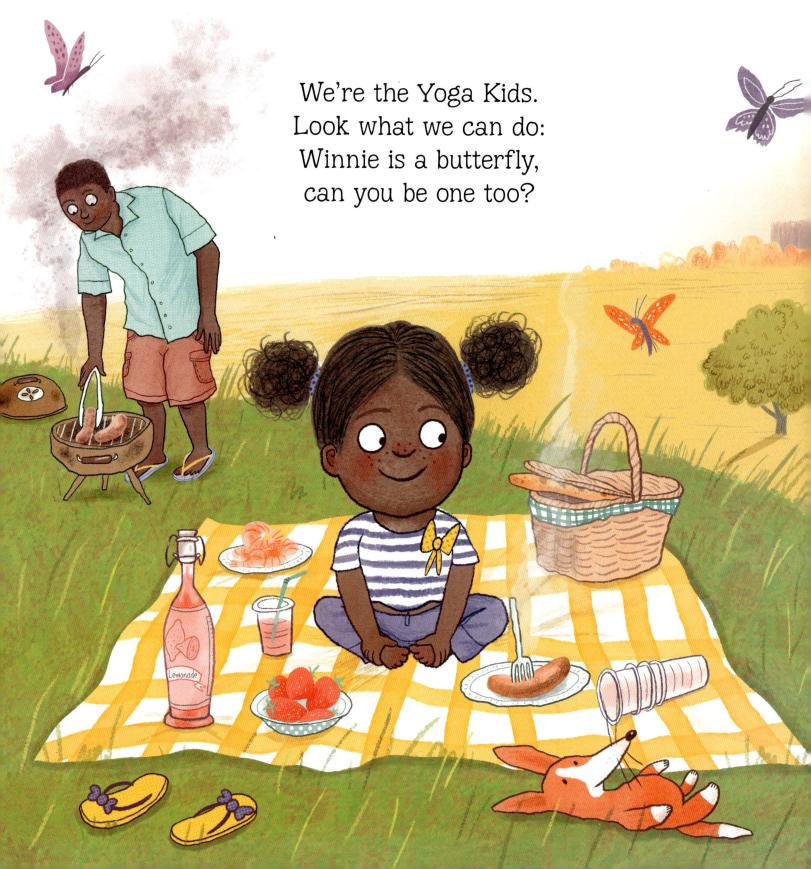

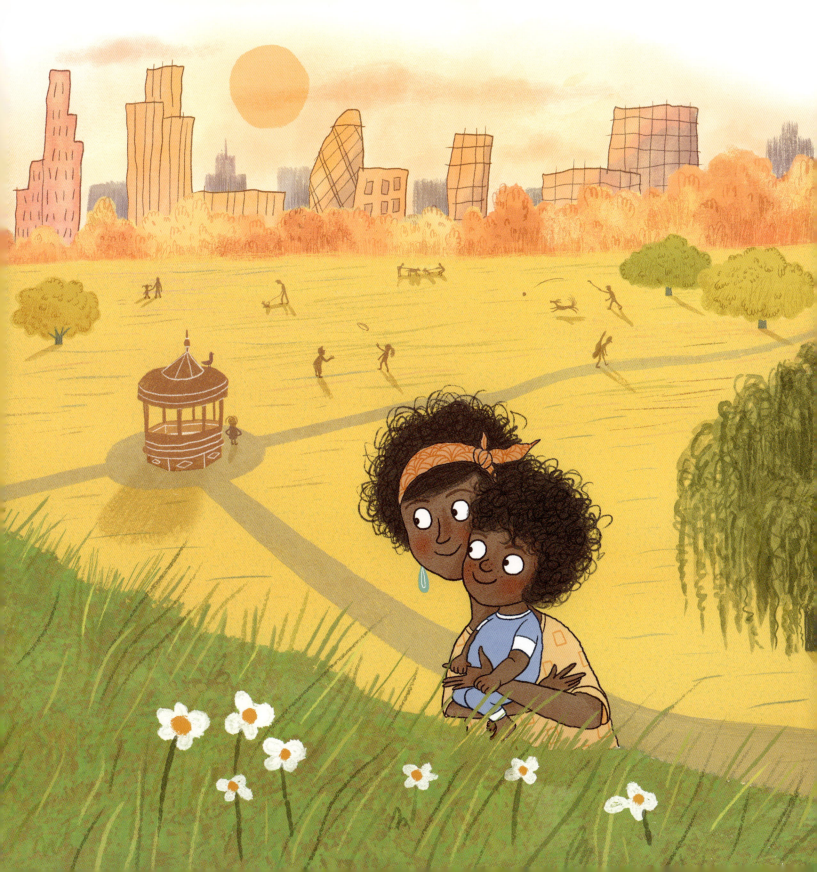

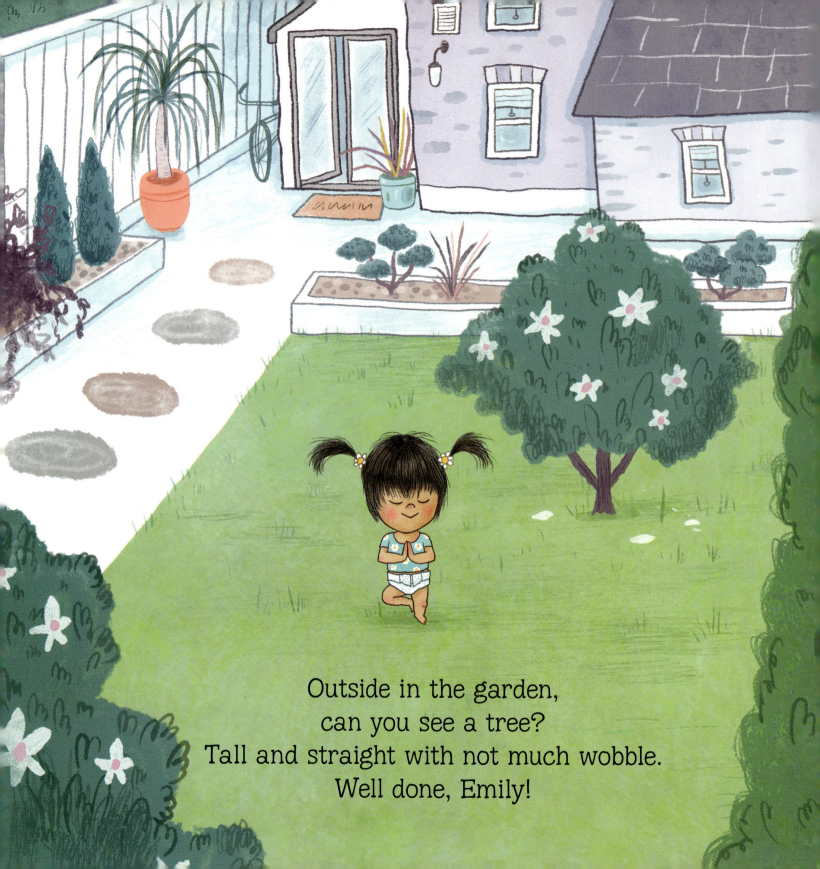

Outside in the garden,
can you see a tree?
Tall and straight with not much wobble.
Well done, Emily!

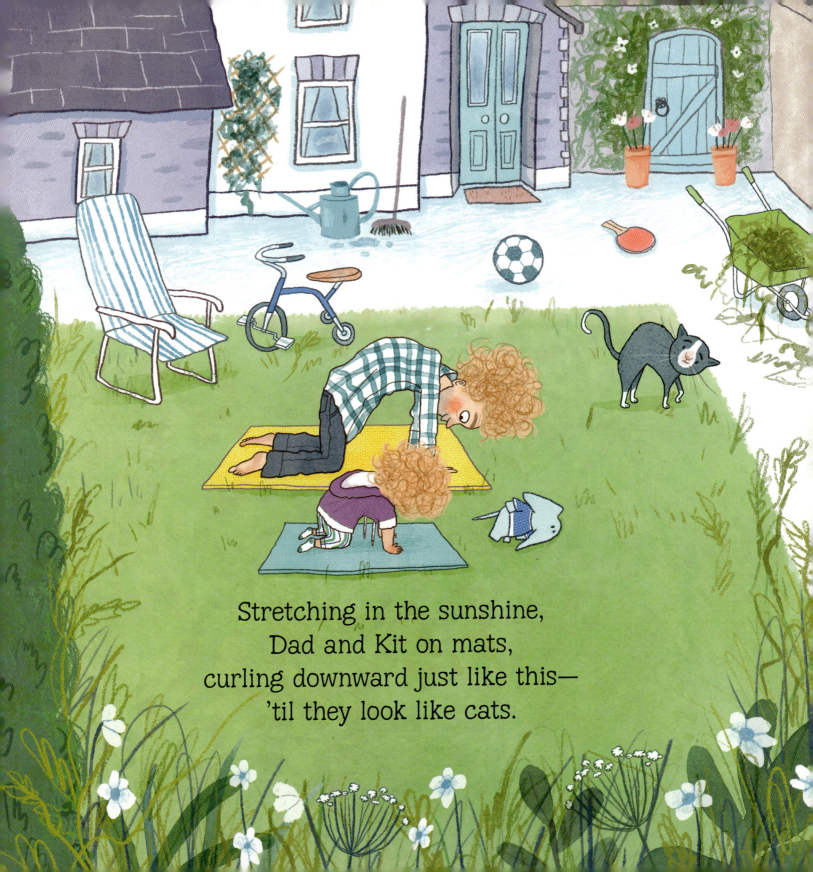

Stretching in the sunshine,
Dad and Kit on mats,
curling downward just like this—
'til they look like cats.

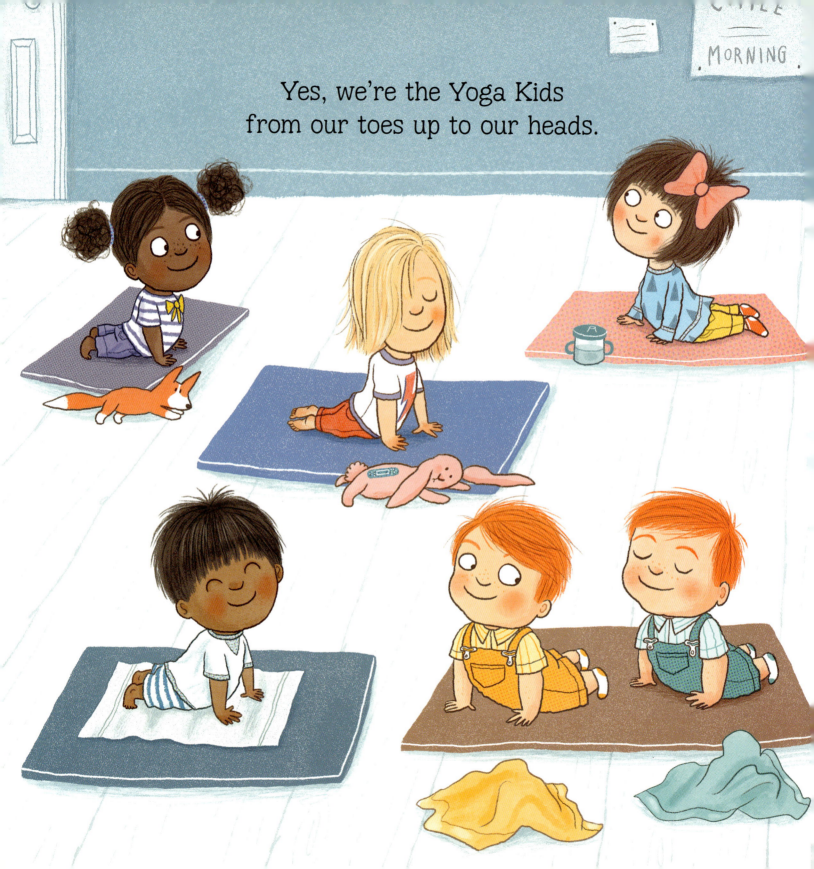
Yes, we're the Yoga Kids from our toes up to our heads.

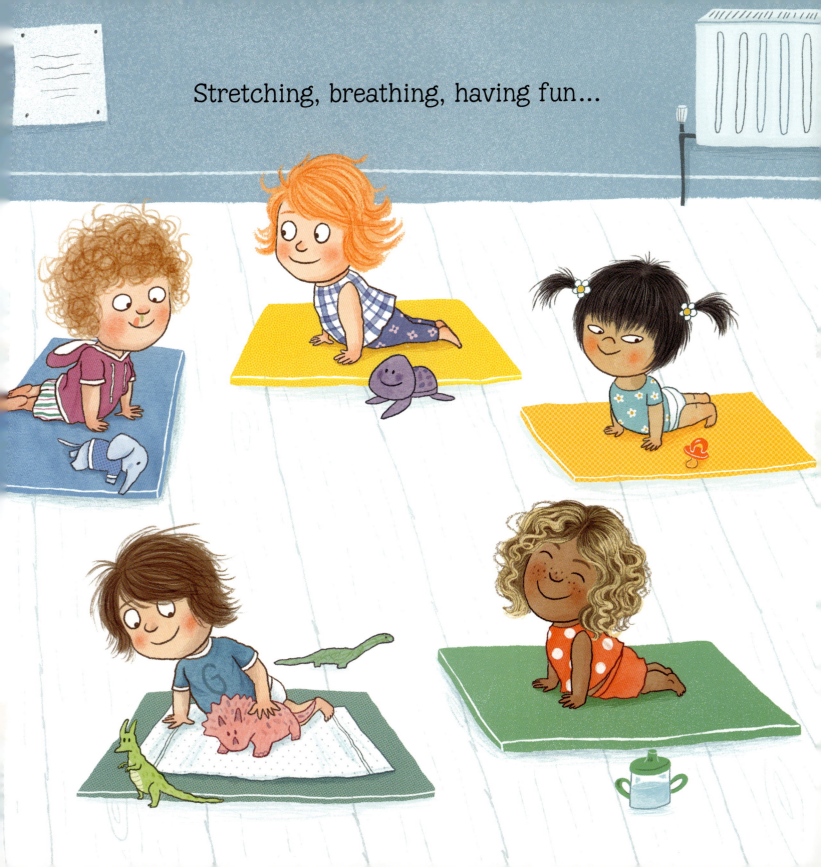
Stretching, breathing, having fun...

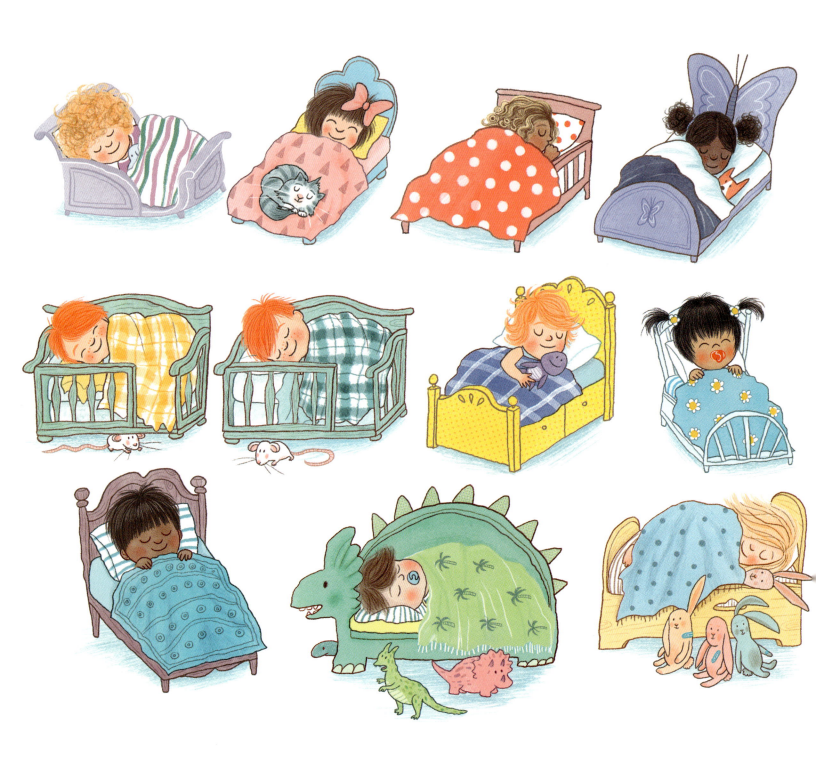

...then snuggling in our beds.

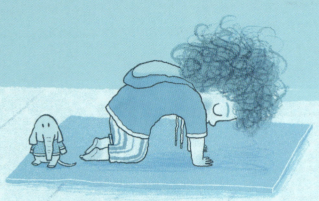
Cat Pose

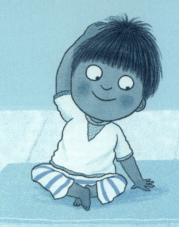
Rainbow Pose

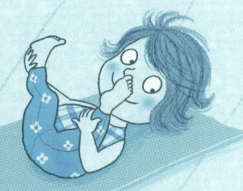
Happy Baby Pose

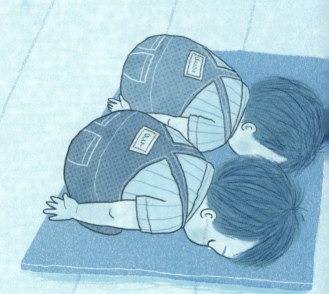
Dormouse Pose

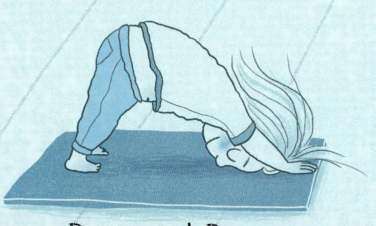
Downward Dog